Carb Cycling for Weight Loss

A Beginner's 3-Week Guide With Sample Curated Recipes

Disclaimer

By reading this disclaimer, you are accepting the terms of the disclaimer in full. If you disagree with this disclaimer, please do not read the guide. The content in this guide is provided for informational and educational purposes only.

This guide is not intended to be a substitute for the original work of this diet plan. At most, this guide is intended to be a beginner's supplement to the original work for this diet plan and never act as a direct substitute. This guide is an overview, review, and commentary on the facts of that diet plan. All product names, diet plans, or names used in this guide are for identification purposes only and are the property of their respective owners. The use of these names does not imply endorsement. All other trademarks cited herein are the property of their respective owners.

None of the information in this guide should be accepted as independent medical or other professional advice. The information in the guide has been compiled from various sources that are deemed reliable. It has been analyzed and summarized to the best of the Author's ability, knowledge, and belief. However, the Author cannot guarantee the accuracy and thus should not be held liable for any errors.

You acknowledge and agree that the Author of

this guide will not be held liable for any damages, costs, expenses, resulting from the application of the information in this book, whether directly or indirectly.

You acknowledge and agree that you assume all risk and responsibility for any action you undertake in response to the information in this guide.

You acknowledge and agree that by continuing to read this guide, you will (where applicable, appropriate, or necessary) consult a qualified medical professional on this information.

The information in this guide is not intended to be any sort of medical advice and should not be used in lieu of any medical advice by a licensed and qualified medical professional.

Always seek the advice of your physician or another qualified health provider with any issues or questions you might have regarding any sort of medical condition. Do not ever disregard any qualified professional medical advice or delay seeking that advice because of anything you have read in this guide.

Table of Contents

Introduction

Do you want to lose weight quickly while still enjoying the carbs you intake? If yes, you're in the right place to learn how.

By its definition, carb cycling is another process of reducing fats and maintaining physical fitness by altering your carb intake. It is a dietary method that can be modified as a daily, weekly, or monthly plan. Moreover, carb cycling's main goal is to organize carbohydrate intake when it delivers extreme advantage and remove it when it is not needed.

Carb cycling is ideal for bodybuilders and other high-performing athletes, but it can also be used by people who want to become physically fit.

Experts even argue that carb cycling can be more effective for most people who want to lose weight because of how it can be easily modified to adapt to a specific lifestyle. It also aims to make sure that you're getting the right amount of nutrients and calories based on your body weight.

It's a relatively new type of dietary plan that still needs more scientific research to back up its effects, but because it greatly supports the consumption of the right calories and nutrients needed per individual, it's still considered a relatively safe diet program to try out, especially if you want to lose weight without too much food restrictions.

In this short guide, you will discover:
- What carb cycling is
- How carb cycling works
- Benefits of carb cycling
- Weight loss in carb cycling
- How to plan your carb cycling journey

Chapter I: All about Carb Cycling

Carb cycling is a dietary plan that involves planned alternations of carb intake. It's meant to consistently provide carbohydrates in your diet but divided into two parts—low carb and high carb—alternating between the two types of carbohydrates—simple and complex carbohydrates.

Carbohydrates are a good source of calories and nutrients. Carb cycling is a great diet program that doesn't cut out carb consumption, but is still effective and is a great program, especially for those who want to lose fat, increase muscle mass, or store carbs for long-haul exercises and workouts, particularly for serious athletes and weightlifters. That was what Franco Carlotto, a 6-time Mr. World Fitness Champion, had in mind when he created this carb cycling program.

In consuming carbohydrates, the body breaks them down into glucose, which is used as fuel for the body. When you're more active, say for days when you need to exercise, you need more fuel for your body. However, when you have a sedentary lifestyle or you don't work out as much, consuming high carbs may lead to weight gain, or worse, diabetes, as glucose turns into stored fats.

With carb cycling, you can properly schedule the days when you must consume high and low carbs. On tough workout days, consume high carbs to ensure you have enough energy as you work out. For your rest days, you also have to take a break from high carb consumption, thus switching to a low carb diet. Your body then uses up the stored fats to burn as fuel, aiding you to lose weight.

Benefits of Carb Cycling
Scientifically, it is yet to be proven how beneficial carb cycling is for health, most especially in the long run. However, its principles align with how healthy eating is encouraged for most people. While it still requires controlled studies to prove these health benefits, here are some known benefits of this program as backed up by other similar diet and workout programs that go well with carb cycling:

- Weight and Fat Loss
  In carb cycling, the goal is to teach your body to adapt to carbohydrate manipulation through controlled or patterned carbohydrate consumption. This promotes calories deficit in the body which then results in weight loss as the body burns stored fats to use as body fuel.

- Muscle Gain
  If you're an athlete or a fan of extreme workouts, carb cycling is a good way to develop your muscles. Muscle-building workouts require great power, you can get

enough energy to do this when you consume high carbs.

- Improvement on the Body
It is believed that a low carbohydrate intake improves insulin sensitivity and cholesterol levels. It also helps in enhancing the body's metabolism.

  During high carbohydrate refeed, the diet helps in enhancing some hormones like the thyroid hormones, testosterone, and leptin, aiding in metabolism, hunger, and workout performance.

Is Carb Cycling Safe?
Carb cycling is safe as long as you consult first with your doctor and you follow the diet protocols. It doesn't necessarily restrict your diet but aids in making you consume the right amount of calories based on your lifestyle. It's important to make sure this is well planned out or you might end up getting sick. For example, if you take low to moderate-carbs and do excessive work, you might experience unusual fatigue. Engaging in low-carbohydrates intake during a workout period may cause stress, fatigue, and may also lead to serious illness because of a lack of energy fuel.

Another piece of advice by carb cycling users is to take note of how your body reacts to this diet program. If you're doing it right but are feeling fatigued, bloated, constipated, or having problems with sleep, you're most likely experiencing carb flu. Staying hydrated by drinking water and electrolytes will help.

How to Start Carb Cycling

Carb cycling is an effective diet when it's done properly. Firstly, you can start it off by making meal plans, listing the foods to take during high, moderate, and low carbohydrates days. Secondly, think about the number of meals that you'd take in a day. Lastly, monitor your diet routine and record its effects weekly to help you keep track of how your body reacts to this program.

There are different variations to carb cycling. It depends on what's best for your body and your ultimate goals. It can be in the form of a 7-day meal plan where you take high-carbs and low-carbs alternately. This style is good for women who want to try out carb cycling.

Other than that, you can try a longer period of the high and low-carbs cycle. This will be highly dependent on your planned physical activities for the day. During your training or heavy workout days, make sure the meals you planned are high in carbohydrates, so your body will have enough energy fuel to keep you going. During your rest days, your meal plans should be low in carbohydrates and rich in protein and fat. This way, you'll still provide additional fuel to your body while it burns stored fats to keep you moving and going about your daily life.

You can also try a longer period of low-carb intake, followed by a shorter period of high-carb intake called refeeding. After a long duration of a strict diet, reward yourself by refeeding. Then, go back to strict dieting to burn the fats that you stored during refeeding.

Take note that you can effectively modify your carb cycling meal plan if you think your body isn't adapting well to the program. However, it's important to remember that due to the lack of scientific studies that tackle its effectiveness, benefits, and risks most especially in the long run, it's highly advised that strict carb cycling be followed only for a short period.

Chapter II: Losing Weight through Carb Cycling

Different diet regimens are designed to help achieve different goals and meet varying needs. Carb cycling specifically meets the needs of high-performing athletes and bodybuilders that need to build muscles and maintain their body fat. However, this doesn't mean ordinary people can't try this program. Because it doesn't specifically restrict you from eating what you normally consume, it's a diet program that can be adapted based on your needs. If your goal is to lose weight without totally giving up on what you love to eat, carb cycling may be a good diet program for you to try.

When you follow the carb cycling program aiming to lose weight, be reminded that you can modify it according to your daily activities. Doing so will make the program more effective, especially if you do it with a regular workout routine, no matter the intensity. Normally, a week of carb cycling diet consists of the high-moderate-low phases: two days of high carbs, two days of moderate carbs, and three days of low carbs.

How Weight Loss Happens in Carb Cycling

Carb cycling is similar to how the ketogenic diet aids in weight loss—because the diet is consumed only of low carbs, the body can burn stored fats to use as fuel. During the low carb phase of this plan, it gives the body the same opportunity to burn stored body fats as you take a break from consuming a high carb diet.

As experts explained, carb cycling is a more advanced diet strategy compared to most diet programs because it requires more programming of the body depending on the set activities, and manipulation of carb benefits depending on your needs during those activities. It's also more focused on ensuring that your calorie consumption is enough based on your age, height, and weight.

According to experts, a healthy basis for sources of daily calories should be broken down into the following: 50 to 55% must come from carbohydrates, 10 to 15% from proteins, and less than 28% from fats. Just remember, daily calorie requirement is not one-size-fits-all information, so make sure you consult with your doctor or research on this first to find out your specific daily caloric needs.

During the high carb days, usually two days of the week, you have to include an exercise or workout program to burn the calories you're consuming. Otherwise, these calories will then be stored as fats.

For your moderate and low carb days, you may consider this as your normal routine days, minus the more intensive workout routine but still taking the time to move around, doing chores or work. If you're able to do a light-intensity workout during these days, all the better.

There are several factors that you can follow as a basis for curating your own carb cycling program, one of which is the popular approach as mentioned before—higher carb consumption on workout days and lower carb consumption on rest days. Another factor you may also want to consider is by basing your cycle on your body fat. Meaning, you add high carb days to your program as you lose weight to help you build stamina and muscles when you work out.

Carb Cycling for Women
To ensure an effective weight loss carb cycling program for women, it is best that you do it daily, alternating on a high carb and low carb diet. Does this mean you have to exercise at least 3 or 4 times a week as well? That depends on you, but of course highly encouraged to help your body burn the calories effectively. It doesn't have to be an intensive workout, but you have to be consistent in staying active especially during your high carb days.

This diet program is also commonly used by those who have encountered weight loss plateau. This is extremely relatable to women, as hormone changes usually affect the body majorly. Women are also prone to having water weight, especially before the menstrual cycle. When you take control of what you eat and base the number of calories you consume on the days when you can burn these calories through intense workouts, this will help your body get back in weight loss mode.

Just a reminder though. If you're pregnant and/or breastfeeding, you should not try this diet. The same goes for those who are underweight and are managing an eating disorder, whether in the present or the past.

Chapter III: Prepping for the Journey

Before diving into this journey, make sure that you have first consulted with your doctor about your plan. It's also necessary that you check the appropriate caloric intake that's exactly what your body needs. This is where carb cycling calculators will come in handy. These types of calculators will help you determine the proper caloric intake based on your age, gender, height, weight, and level of activity. It's extremely helpful, especially if you're still navigating through this diet program. Having the right information will make this program much more effective and will have you successfully achieve your goals.

There are two common methods in doing carb cycling, according to Fitness Coach JC Deen. He also mentioned that there is not a right way to do carb cycling, but planning out your meal plan will be a great help to keep you on track. Here are the two methods that you can start with:

- High/Low Method – Alternating days of high carb and low carb. A high carb day must cover at least 150 grams of carbohydrates intake while a low carb day must cover at most 100 grams of carbohydrates intake.

- High/Moderate/Low Method – Alternating days of high, moderate, and low carb. A high carb day must cover at least 150 grams of carbohydrates intake, a medium carb day must cover between 100-150 grams of carbohydrates intake, while a low carb day must cover at most 100 grams of carbohydrates intake.

In addition to identifying the methods, you can also curate your carb cycling plan on the type you want to focus on, either for fat loss or muscle gain. When you opt for fat loss carb cycling, you'll be training your body to burn consumed carbs and stored body fats. Because you're limiting the consumption of carbs, you are placing yourself in what is called a caloric deficit. As for those who want to gain muscle, they undergo what is called a caloric surplus, which aids in recovery during training days and also helps in the growth of more muscle tissues.

As for exercises and workouts, you can choose the ones that will work best with your lifestyle. There are a lot of varying intensity workouts that can be as short as 7 minutes. If you're someone who can't do intense workouts, a simple walk or jog to the park for around half an hour at least can be a good workout routine to pair with your carb cycling plan. As you become more accustomed to the routine and the program, you can also level up on the physical activities, especially when you start to shed some pounds.

It is also recommended to keep a diary to document your daily experiences while doing this diet program. This will greatly be useful when you need to identify certain aspects of your meal plan that were effective or problematic, depending on how your body reacted. This will also be extremely useful for your doctor to review on your next visit.

Chapter IV: Carb Cycling Week One

Now that it's the first week of your carb cycling journey, you may either experience it differently or not, depending on how your body will react. Just make sure that you're following the plan closely and you stay hydrated. Also, try not to go all out at once on your workout plans. Taking things slowly but surely is much more reliable than starting this too enthusiastically. As for the weekly meal plans, here are two types you can use as a guide as you curate your first week. Remember, you may modify these in your next weeks, just ensure that you're sticking to the right daily caloric intake and your new routine:

Days	Exercise	Carb Intake	Fat Intake	Carbs in Grams
1, 3, 5, 7	Weight Training or Aerobic Exercise	High Carb	Low Fat	Not less than 150g*
2, 4, 6	Rest	Low Carb	High Fat	Not more than 100g*

*from jcdfitness.com[1]

[1] https://jcdfitness.com/2017/09/carb-cycling-meal-plan/

Here's another one for the High/Mod/Low Carb meal plan:

Day	Exercise	Carb Intake	Fat Intake	Carbs in Grams
1	Weight Training	High Carb	Low Fat	200g
2	Aerobic Exercise	Mod Carb	Mod Fat	100g
3	Rest Day	Low Carb	High Fat	30g
4	Weight Training	High Carb	Low Fat	200g
5	Weight Training	High Carb	Low Fat	200g
6	Rest	Low Carb	High Fat	30g
7	Rest	Low Carb	High Fat	30g

Sample High/Mod/Low Carb meal plan from healthline.com[2]

The sample meal plans don't show the recommended daily nutrients you need to aid you in your diet, but you'll need them especially during your rest days. Protein can be an essential agent to aid in weight loss through soothing blood sugar and sustaining muscle mass. Fiber supports the regulation of blood sugar, which is necessary to maintain regular body weight. To improve body composition, you need to include around 3-6 grams of omega 3 fatty acids during your meals. Staying hydrated is also extremely important, especially when you experience carb fever a few days into your diet.

As for food restrictions, there are still a few, which can easily be substituted with better,

---

[2]   https://www.healthline.com/nutrition/carb-cycling-101#TOC_TITLE_HDR_7

healthier options. Avoid drinking flavored beverages as they contain unhealthy carbs and may become a hindrance to your progress. Opt for water and natural teas instead. Stay away from condiments such as ketchup and salad dressings as they also contain a high amount of carbohydrates. Spices are better alternatives for the usual condiments.

Chapter V: Carb Cycling Week Two

For the second week, you have most likely adjusted to the carb cycling diet. You will be tempted to break from your diet and try out some food you might be missing, but remember, consistency is key. Drinking water or tea will help ease food cravings.

The first week was all about introducing your body to the diet, gradually programming your body to burn calories and stored fats depending on the day. As for the second week, it's a continuation of what you have done so far. You may level up on the exercise you're doing, whether increasing the time you spend on it or the intensity of the workout, or trying out a new routine.

You may also want to try adapting the intermittent fasting routine. According to research, eating meals within an 8 to 10-hour gap burns more fatty acids, enhances insulin sensitivity, and reduces damaged cells. If you want and can, you may also want to try this alongside your carb cycling program. Just make sure you consult first with your doctor.

Week 2 guide:

Day	Exercise	Carb Intake	Fat Intake	Carbs in Grams
1	Weight Training	High Carb	Low Fat	250g
2	Aerobic Exercise	Mod Carb	Mod Fat	150g
3	Weight Training	High Carb	High Fat	250g
4	Rest Day	No Carb	Low Fat	0g
5	Aerobic Exercise	Mod Carb	Mod Fat	150g
6	Rest	Low Carb	High Fat	100g
7	Rest	Low Carb	High Fat	100g

Chapter VI: Carb Cycling Week Three

In your third week, you can level up on the workout routines by choosing higher intensity workouts or doing prolonged routines. You're more likely used to modifying your meals now, substituting for healthier options even during your high/moderate carb days.

Week 3 guide:

Day	Exercise	Carb Intake	Fat Intake	Carbs in Grams
1	Weight Training	High Carb	Low Fat	250g
2	Aerobic Exercise	Mod Carb	Mod Fat	150g
3	Rest Day	No Carb	High Fat	0g
4	Weight Training	High Carb	Low Fat	250g
5	Aerobic Exercise	Mod Carb	Mod Fat	150g
6	Rest	Low Carb	High Fat	100g
7	Rest	No Carb	High Fat	0g

Take note that while it is advised that you do this diet program for only a short time if you think doing the carb cycling greatly benefitted your health and want to continue doing the program, make sure that you consult first with your doctor, and allow them to assess your health post-carb cycling.

Chapter VI: Carb Cycling Recipes

Here are some healthy high and low-carb recipes you can follow during your carb cycling journey.

Healthy High Carb Recipes

Carrot Cake Oats

Ingredients:
- 1/2 cup dry oats cooked with water
- 1 scoop vanilla whey protein powder
- 3 oz. unsweetened almond milk
- 2-3 tbsp. grated carrots
- allspice, to taste
- cinnamon, to taste
- nutmeg, to taste
- 1 tbsp. maple syrup
- Optional: 1 tbsp. sliced almonds
- Optional: 1 tbsp. shaved coconut

Instructions:
1. Cook up some oats using water and set them aside.
2. In a shaker bottle, mix almond milk and protein powder vigorously until well-mixed. Add to the serving of oatmeal and mix.
3. Add the remaining ingredients. Stir well.
4. Serve as is or warm up the oatmeal in the microwave before serving.

Chicken and Broccoli Casserole

Ingredients:
- ☐ 1 tbsp. olive oil
- ☐ 1 tbsp. garlic, minced
- ☐ 1/2 red onion, diced
- ☐ 1 cup uncooked brown rice
- ☐ 1 tsp. thyme
- ☐ 1 tsp. rosemary
- ☐ 3-1/2 cups low sodium chicken broth
- ☐ 1 lb. chicken breast, chopped into 1-inch pieces
- ☐ 1/2 cup (4 oz.) 2% Greek yogurt
- ☐ 2/3 cup 3-cheese blend
- ☐ 12 oz. raw broccoli florets

Instructions:
1. Set the slow cooker to low heat sauté function.
2. Sauté olive oil, garlic, and onion until the onions caramelize.
3. Add uncooked brown rice, fresh rosemary, and fresh thyme.
4. Mix well. Ensure that rice is well-covered with the seasoning.
5. Pour in chicken broth followed by diced raw chicken breasts.
6. Stir and pop the top. Cook on medium-high heat for 3 to 5 hours.

7. An hour before the cooking time ends, mix it again and add Greek yogurt and cheese. Mix it until creamy.
8. Place raw broccoli florets on top of the rice.
9. Season to taste with sea salt & pepper.

Sweet Potato Salad

Ingredients:
- ☐ 3 large sweet potatoes, peeled
- ☐ 1 red bell pepper, diced
- ☐ 2 celery stalks, chopped
- ☐ 1/2 medium red onion, diced

Sauce:
- ☐ 1/4 cup safflower mayo
- ☐ 2 heaping tbsp. 2% Greek yogurt
- ☐ 1 tbsp. Dijon mustard
- ☐ 1 tsp. smoked paprika
- ☐ cumin, to taste
- ☐ fresh orange juice
- ☐ sea salt, to taste
- ☐ pepper, to taste
- ☐ Optional: 1 tsp. fresh rosemary
- ☐ Optional: a pinch of turmeric

Garnish:
- ☐ fresh chopped green onion
- ☐ 1/2 cup goat cheese crumble, may adjust the amount to taste

Instructions:
1. Boil sweet potatoes until tender, about 12-15 minutes. Strain and set aside to cool down.

2. In a bowl, mix the ingredients for the sauce. Season to taste with sea salt & pepper.
3. Chop the sweet potato into chunks.
4. In a large bowl, add the sweet potato and chopped veggies, top with the sauce. Gently fold the ingredients together.
5. Serve warm or chilled.

Chicken Wrap (Cajun Style)

Ingredients:
- Keto tortilla
- Avocado, half will do, chopped
- Cajun chicken
- Tomato, chopped
- Yogurt, preferably plain or organic, to taste
- Lettuce, chopped
- Cucumber, chopped
- Pepper, to taste
- Sea salt, to taste

Instructions:
1. Except for the tortilla, toss all the ingredients for the salad in a bowl.
2. Heat the tortilla in the microwave for 15 seconds, then plate it nicely.

3. Gently transfer the salad mix to the center of the tortilla. Once done, fold both sides nicely, similar to how a burrito is wrapped.
4. Slice and enjoy eating.

Egg Salad with Avocados

Ingredients:

- [ ] 3 medium-sized avocados
- [ ] 6 eggs, large and hard-boiled
- [ ] 1/3 red onion, medium size
- [ ] 3 celery ribs
- [ ] 4 tbsps. Mayonnaise
- [ ] 2 tbsps. Freshly squeezed lime juice
- [ ] 2 tsp. brown mustard
- [ ] 1/2 tsp. cumin powder
- [ ] 1 tsp. hot sauce
- [ ] Salt and pepper

Instructions:

1. Chop the eggs, celery, and onion.
2. Set aside the avocados, then combine the rest of the ingredients.
3. Slice avocado in half to take out the pit.
4. Stuff the avocado by spooning the egg salad on its cave.
5. Serve and enjoy.

Healthy Low Carb Recipes

<u>Roasted Veggies</u>

Ingredients:
- ☐ 1/2 lb. turnips
- ☐ 1/2 lb. carrots
- ☐ 1/2 lb. parsnips
- ☐ 2 shallots, peeled
- ☐ 1/4 tsp. ground black pepper
- ☐ 1 tbsps. extra-virgin olive oil
- ☐ 6 cloves garlic
- ☐ 3/4 tsp. kosher salt
- ☐ 2 tbsp. fresh rosemary needles

Instructions:
1. First, cut vegetables into bite-sized pieces.
2. Set the oven to 400°F.
3. Mix all the ingredients in a baking dish.
4. Roast the vegetables for 25 minutes until brown and tender.
5. Toss and roast again for 20- 25 minutes.
6. Serve and enjoy while hot.

Keto Zucchini Walnut Bread

Ingredients:
- 3 large eggs
- 1/2 cup virgin olive oil
- 1 tsp. vanilla extract
- 2-1/4 cups fine almond flour
- 1-1/2 cups sweetener, erythritol
- 1/2 tsp. salt
- 1-1/2 tsp. baking powder
- 1/2 tsp. nutmeg, ground
- 1 tsp. cinnamon, ground
- 1/4 tsp. ginger, ground
- 1 cup zucchini, grated
- 1/2 cup walnuts, chopped

Instructions:
1. Preheat your oven to 350°F.
2. Whisk together the eggs, oil, and vanilla extract. Set aside.
3. Using another bowl, combine the baking powder, sweetener, almond flour, salt, cinnamon, nutmeg, and ginger powder. Set aside.
4. Squeeze the excess water from the zucchini using a paper towel or a cheesecloth.
5. Pour the zucchini into the egg mixture and whisk.
6. Add the flour mixture slowly into the egg and zucchini mixture. Blend using an

electric blender until the mixture turns smooth.

7. Spray a loaf pan with avocado oil or baking spray.

8. Pour the zucchini batter into the loaf pan and smoothen the top evenly.

9. Spoon the chopped walnuts on top of the batter, lightly pressing the walnuts with the back of a spoon to press into the batter.

10. Pop the loaf pan into the oven and then bake for 60-70 minutes, or until the walnuts turn brown.

11. Cool in a cooling rack before slicing and serving.

Tangy Lemon Fish

Ingredients:
- [ ] 200 g. Gurnard fresh fish fillets
- [ ] 3 tbsp. butter
- [ ] 1 tbsp. fresh lemon juice
- [ ] 1/4 cup fine almond flour
- [ ] 1 tsp. dried dill
- [ ] 1 tsp. dried chives
- [ ] 1 tsp. onion powder
- [ ] 1/2 tsp. garlic powder
- [ ] salt, to taste
- [ ] pepper, to taste

Instructions:
1. On a large plate or tray, combine dill, almond flour, and spices. Mix until well combined.
2. Dredge each fillet one at a time into the flour mix. Turn the fillet around until fully coated, and then transfer to a clean plate or tray. This may be refrigerated until ready to cook.
3. Place a large pan over medium-high heat.
4. Combine halves of butter and lemon juice. Swirl the pan to mix, lift occasionally to avoid burning the butter.
5. Allow the fish to cook for about 3 minutes.
6. Let the fish absorb all the lemony-butter mixture. Cook on low heat to avoid drying out the pan.

7. Add the remaining lemon juice and butter to the pan.
8. Turn the fish to cook the other side for 3 minutes more. Swirl around the pan to fully coat it with the juice.
9. Wait until it turns golden brown and the fish is cooked through.
10.   Serve with buttered vegetables.

Spinach and Watercress Salad

Ingredients:

- 1 cup watercress, washed with stems removed
- 3 cups baby spinach, washed with stems removed
- 1 medium sliced avocado
- 1/4 cup avocado oil
- 1/8 cup lemon juice
- a pinch of salt

Instructions:

1. Pat dry the spinach and watercress. Remove the stem and separate the leaves.
2. On a large serving plate, combine the leaves of the watercress and the spinach.
3. Cut the avocado in half then remove the pit. Peel the skin off from each side.
4. Slice the avocadoes into thin strips. Set aside.
5. Prepare the dressing by combining avocado oil and lemon juice.
6. Arrange the avocado strips on top of the watercress and spinach.
7. Season with salt and pepper.
8. Drizzle with the dressing before serving.

Baked Salmon

Ingredients:
- 2 salmon fillets
- 6 cups of fresh spinach
- 2 tsp. coconut oil
- 1 tsp. coconut oil
- 1/4 tsp. garlic powder
- 1/4 tsp. turmeric
- 3 large cloves of garlic
- lemon juice
- salt and pepper, to taste

Instructions:
1. Preheat the oven to 400°F.
2. Line a baking dish with parchment paper.
3. Marinate salmon fillets in lemon juice, coconut oil, garlic powder, turmeric, salt, and pepper.
4. Let it sit for a few minutes. This may also be done the night before to help the juices and flavor get into the salmon.
5. Once the oven is ready, bake salmon for 15 minutes.
6. Cook some of the garlic in a pan with coconut oil.
7. Add spinach and cook until ready. Season with salt and pepper to taste.
8. Take salmon out of the oven and put spinach beside.

9. Serve and enjoy.

Lemon Roasted Broccoli

Ingredients:
- [ ] 1-1/2 lb. broccoli florets
- [ ] 1/3 cup shredded Parmesan cheese
- [ ] 1/4 cup olive oil
- [ ] 2 tbsps. fresh basil, chopped
- [ ] 3 tsp. minced garlic
- [ ] 1/2 – 3/4 tsp. kosher salt
- [ ] 1/2 tsp. red chili flakes
- [ ] 1/2 lemon juice and zest

Instructions:
1. Preheat the oven to 425°F.
2. Line a baking sheet with parchment paper and spread the broccoli florets.
3. Season the broccoli with basil, olive oil, garlic, kosher salt, chili flakes, lemon zest, and lemon juice.
4. Sprinkle the top with parmesan cheese then put into the oven for 20-25 minutes or until the cheese has slightly melted.
5. Serve and enjoy while warm.

Flat Bread

Ingredients:
- 1/2 cup coconut flour
- 1 tbsp. ground psyllium husk powder
- 1/4 cup olive oil
- 1 cup boiling water
- 1/3 cup grated parmesan cheese or mozzarella cheese
- 1/2 tsp. sea salt
- 1/4 tsp. granulated garlic
- 1/2 tbsp. black peppercorns
- 1/2 tbsp. rosemary, dried

Instructions:
1. Whisk all the dry ingredients together in a mixing bowl.
2. Add olive oil and cheese.
3. While stirring, add the hot water. Continue to stir until the psyllium fiber and coconut flour have absorbed all of the water.
4. Flatten the dough onto parchment paper on a baking sheet, until it is 1/8-inch thin and even.
5. Bake for 20-25 minutes. Baking time will depend on the thickness of the dough.
6. When browned, transfer to a cooling rack, peel away the parchment paper, and allow the flatbread to cool.
7. Use a pizza cutter to cut the flatbread into squares for sandwiches.

8. Store any leftovers in the refrigerator.

Stuffed Chicken

Ingredients:
- 4 pcs. Foster Farm's chicken breast fillets, skinless and boneless
- 1/4 cup feta cheese, crumbled
- 1/4 cup artichoke hearts, finely chopped, drained and marinated
- 2 tbsp. red peppers, finely chopped, drained, and roasted
- 2 tbsp. green onion, thinly sliced
- 2 tsp. fresh oregano, or 1/2 tsp. if using dried oregano
- 1 tsp. kosher salt
- 1/4 tsp. ground black pepper

Instructions:
1. Cut a pocket in each chicken breast using a sharp knife. Cut through the thickest portion horizontally without cutting through the opposite side.
2. Combine into a mixture the feta, roasted peppers, artichoke hearts, oregano, and green onions.
3. Fill each pocket of the chicken breast with the mixture.
4. Close the opening of the pockets with a wooden toothpick.
5. Season the chicken breast with salt and pepper.

6. Preheat a non-stick large skillet on medium heat.
7. Coat it with cooking spray.
8. Fry the chicken for 10 to 12 minutes on each side, or until the internal temperature reaches at least 165°F.
9. Serve hot.

Grilled Lamb

Ingredients:
- ☐ 1-1/2 lb. baby spinach leaves
- ☐ 3 tbsp. dried oregano, chopped
- ☐ 1/4 cup lemon juice
- ☐ 1/4 cup olive oil
- ☐ 2 tbsp. ground cumin
- ☐ 1 tsp. crushed red pepper
- ☐ 1 tbsp. coarse sea salt
- ☐ 1 tbsp. squeezed juice from an orange
- ☐ 3 cloves garlic
- ☐ 2 yellow onions, chopped
- ☐ cooking spray

Directions:
1. In a 2-gallon zip bag, put the lamb together with the lemon juice, oregano, cumin, and salt.
2. Close the bag and refrigerate overnight
3. Puree onions, garlic, some orange juice, and olive oil in a blender.
4. Transfer to a small bowl with a cover.
5. Chill overnight.
6. Mix sea salt, red pepper, and cumin in a small bowl
7. Remove refrigerated lamb and let it sit for 30 minutes.
8. Preheat the grill to medium.
9. Place lamb on the grill and coat with some cooking spray or oil.

10. Grill lamb for one and a half hours over medium heat.
11. Remove lamb from the grill.
12. Serve hot.

Ground Beef Stroganoff

Ingredients:
- ☐ 1 lb. 80%
- ☐ lean ground beef
- ☐ 2 tbsp. butter
- ☐ 1 clove garlic, minced
- ☐ 10 oz. sliced mushrooms
- ☐ 1 tbsp. fresh parsley, chopped
- ☐ 1 tbsp. fresh lemon juice
- ☐ salt
- ☐ pepper
- ☐ 2 tbsps. water

Instructions:
1. Heat the large skillet over medium heat.
2. Put in the butter, letting it melt.
3. Add in the garlic and wait until it turns brown
4. Add beef and season with salt and pepper.
5. When the garlic turns brown, add the beef. Season with salt and pepper.
6. Drain some of the oil from the skillet.
7. Add the mushroom to the leftover oil and cook for 2 minutes. Add water.
8. Reduce the heat temperature to low. Add the lemon juice.
9. Garnish with parsley and serve immediately.

Banana Bread

Ingredients:
- [ ] 1 cup olive oil mayonnaise
- [ ] 2 eggs
- [ ] 4 medium ripe bananas
- [ ] 2 tsp. vanilla extract
- [ ] 2 cups unbleached all-purpose flour
- [ ] 1 cup whole wheat flour
- [ ] 3/4 cup Brown Xylitol
- [ ] 2 tsp. baking soda
- [ ] 2 tsp. sea salt
- [ ] 2 tsp. cinnamon
- [ ] 1 tsp. baking powder
- [ ] Optional: nuts, flax, wheat germ, whey protein, whichever you prefer

Instructions:
1. Preheat the oven to 350°F.
2. In a large mixing bowl, mash bananas, mix in mayonnaise, eggs, and vanilla extract.
3. In a separate bowl, combine the remaining dry ingredients.
4. Add the dry ingredients to the wet ingredients.
5. Stir in nuts if desired.
6. Divide the batter into two greased loaf pans.
7. Bake in the center rack of the oven for 45 to 50 minutes.

8. Let stand for 10 minutes. Remove from pan to finish cooling.
9. Serve and enjoy.

Healthy Green Smoothie

Ingredients:
- 1 cup fresh spinach
- 1/2 tsp. mint extract or to taste
- Optional: 1/4 tsp. peppermint liquid Stevia

Instructions:
1. Gather the ingredients.
2. Add them to a high-powered blender.
3. Turn on the blender.
4. Add them to glass and freeze for 5 minutes.
5. Serve and enjoy.

Red Velvet Molten Lava Cake

Ingredients:
- ☐ 2 tbsp. coconut flour
- ☐ 1 tbsp. ground flaxseed meal
- ☐ 1 tbsp. unsweetened cocoa powder
- ☐ 1/4 tsp. salt
- ☐ 1/2 tsp. baking powder
- ☐ 1/4 cup 1% milk
- ☐ 2 eggs
- ☐ 1/4 tsp. vanilla extract
- ☐ 1 tsp. chocolate liquid stevia, or 1/2 cup of sugar-free sweetener
- ☐ 3 drops of red food coloring
- ☐ 85% dark chocolate bars, broken into pieces

Instructions:
1. Whisk the coconut flour, flaxseed, cocoa powder, salt, and baking powder together.
2. In another bowl, whisk together the milk, eggs, vanilla extract, stevia, and food coloring.
3. Add the dry ingredients into the wet and stir until combined.
4. Adjust food coloring to the redness you desire.
5. Spray two ramekins or microwave-safe mugs.
6. Pour batter evenly into each dish.

7. In the center of each batter, insert the broken chocolate pieces.
8. Microwave one cake at a time for about one minute and 30 seconds.
9. Serve and enjoy while warm.

Chicken Masala Crock Pot Style

Ingredients:
- ☐ 6 boneless skinless chicken breasts, halved lengthwise
- ☐ 2 cloves of minced garlic
- ☐ 2 tbsp. extra virgin olive oil
- ☐ 1 tsp. salt
- ☐ 1 tsp. pepper
- ☐ 2 cups Marsala wine or chicken broth
- ☐ 1 cup of cold water
- ☐ 1/2 cup arrowroot powder
- ☐ 16 oz. sliced baby Portobello mushrooms
- ☐ 3 tbsp. fresh parsley, chopped

Instructions:
1. Grease the slow cooker. Add garlic and oil.
2. Season chicken with salt and pepper on each side and lay in the crockpot.
3. Pour wine over chicken and cover the crockpot.
4. Cook on high for 3 hours.
5. Mix water with arrowroot and stir until absorbed.
6. Remove chicken from the crockpot and keep warm.
7. Stir in arrowroot water mixture into the bottom of the crockpot. Add mushrooms.
8. Add back the chicken. Stir well to coat chicken with sauce and mushrooms.
9. Cover and cook for an additional hour.

10.	Serve with a sprinkle of chopped fresh parsley.

Balsamic-Glazed Chicken Thighs

Ingredients:
- 1 tsp. garlic powder
- 1 tsp. dried basil
- 1/2 tsp. salt
- 1/2 tsp. pepper
- 2 tsp. dehydrated onion
- 4 garlic cloves, minced
- 1 tbsp. extra-virgin olive oil
- 1/2 cup balsamic vinegar, divide equally
- 8 chicken thighs, boneless and skinless
- fresh chopped parsley, for garnish

Instructions:
1. Combine the first five dry spices in a small bowl. Spread over chicken on both sides. Set aside.
2. Pour olive oil and garlic on the bottom of the crockpot.
3. Pour in 1/4 cup balsamic vinegar.
4. Place chicken on top.
5. Sprinkle remaining balsamic vinegar over the chicken.
6. Cover and cook on high for 3 hours.
7. Sprinkle fresh parsley on top to serve.

Zero Carb Buttery Noodles

Ingredients:
- ☐ 7 oz. shirataki noodles
- ☐ 2 tbsp. unsalted butter
- ☐ 1 tbsp. grated parmesan
- ☐ salt
- ☐ black pepper
- ☐ fresh basil or parsley

Instructions:
1. Drain and rinse the noodles in cold water.
2. Transfer them to a bowl, and cover with boiling water for 5 minutes.
3. Drain again.
4. In a skillet, melt the butter over medium heat.
5. Add the noodles, and sprinkle in some salt.
6. Sauté for 3-4 minutes until the butter has been absorbed.
7. Add pepper to the noodles, garnished with parmesan and basil or parsley.

Zero Carb Bread

Ingredients:
- 3 eggs
- 3 tbsp. cream cheese at room temperature
- 1/4 tsp. baking powder

Instructions:
1. Preheat the oven to 300°F.
2. Separate the yolk from the egg whites.
3. In one bowl, mix the egg yolks, cream cheese, and honey until smooth.
4. In a second bowl, add baking powder to the whites. Beat the whites with the hand mixer at high speed until they are fluffy.
5. Slowly fold the egg yolk mixture into the egg white mixture. Mix carefully, making sure to not break the fluffiness of the egg whites too much.
6. Do the following as quickly as possible, or the mixture may start melting.
7. Spoon the mixture into 10-12 even rounds onto a lightly greased baking sheet.
8. Bake for 18-20 minutes on the middle rack.
9. Broil for a minute or a minute and a half, cooking the top until they become nice and golden brown.

Zero Carb Pizza Crust

Ingredients:
- ☐ 10 oz. canned chicken
- ☐ 1 oz. grated parmesan cheese
- ☐ 1 large egg

Instructions:
1. Drain the canned chicken thoroughly, getting as much moisture out as possible.
2. Spread chicken on a baking sheet lined with a silicone mat.
3. Bake at 350°F for 10 minutes to dry out the chicken.
4. Once it's done, remove and place in a mixing bowl. Increase the heat of the oven to 500°F.
5. Add cheese and egg to the bowl with chicken and mix.
6. Pour mixture onto a baking sheet lined with a silicone mat.
7. Spread thinly. Place parchment paper on top and use a rolling pin to do so.
8. Optional: With a spatula, press in the edges of the crust to create a ridge, to keep off any topping from falling off.
9. Bake the crust for 8-10 minutes at 500°F.
10. Remove crust from the oven.
11. Add desired toppings and bake for another 6-10 minutes at 500°F. Toppings will dictate final cook time.

12. Remove from the oven and allow to cool for a few minutes.
13. Serve and enjoy.

Conclusion

Carb cycling[3] is a well-defined diet program that caters to the specific needs of people who know exactly what they want and what they need to achieve. Professional and serious athletes and weightlifters do this program because it works for them and allows them to enjoy eating and not dread it. These benefits can also be enjoyed

---

[3] References

https://www.precisionnutrition.com/all-about-carb-cycling
https://legionathletics.com/carb-cycling
https://www.healthline.com/nutrition/carb-cycling-101#section1
https://www.eatthis.com/carb-cycling
https://www.livinghealthy.com/experts/franco-carlotto
https://cyklopedia.cc/cycling-nutrition/carb-cycling-for-women/
https://jcdfitness.com/2019/11/carb-cycling-for-women/
www.healthline.com
www.mymetabolicmeals.com
www.jcdfitness.com
https://www.webmd.com/diet/carb-cycling-overview#1
https://www.medicalnewstoday.com/articles/carb-cycling#carb-cycling
https://health.clevelandclinic.org/what-to-eat-if-youre-carb-cycling/
https://www.shape.com/healthy-eating/diet-tips/what-is-carb-cycling
https://www.health.com/weight-loss/carb-cycling
https://www.womenshealthmag.com/weight-loss/a19975595/carb-cycling-for-weight-loss/
https://www.healthline.com/nutrition/20-reasons-you-are-not-losing-weight
https://jcdfitness.com/2019/11/carb-cycling-for-women/#more-21932
https://jcdfitness.com/2017/09/carb-cycling-meal-plan/
https://jcdfitness.com/calorie-intake-calculator/
https://www.mymetabolicmeals.com/?s=carb+cycling+meal+plan&paged=1

by non-athletic people who are looking to find ways to lose weight, gain muscle mass, or just get motivated to eat healthily.

It's important to take note that while it's a diet program done by high-profile people, carb cycling still lacks scientific depth and research that can further explain or prove its benefits, effectiveness, and risks especially in the longer run. Similar to any diet program, if you wish to give this one a try, make sure you consult first with your doctor to know if your body is ready to take on the journey.

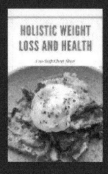

Printed in Great Britain
by Amazon

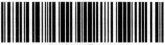

16468842R00038